Vibrant Vitality

A Comprehensive Guide to Healthful Living and Nutritious Eating

By

R. C. Gilbert

Copyright

3
Vibrant vitality

Table of contents

Introduction

· Welcome to Vibrant Vitality

· Navigating the path to well-being

Chapter 1: Foundations of Vibrant Living

· Understanding Holistic Health

· The Interconnectedness of mind, body, and soul

· Setting the stage for lasting vitality

Chapter 2: Nutrition Wisdom

· Macronutrients and micronutrients: The Essentials

· Building a well-balanced plate

· Unmasking Nutrition myths and fads

Chapter 3: Mindful eating

· The art of mindful consumption

· Cultivating a healthy relationship with food

· Savoring the flavor: mindful eating practices

Chapter 4: Holistic Health Practices

· Exercise for energy and well-being

· Stress management strategies

· Quality sleep: The foundation of vitality

Chapter 5: Recipes for Wellness

· Energizing Breakfasts

· Nourishing Lunches and dinners

· Irresistible snacks and smoothies

Chapter 6: Lifestyle Strategies

· Time management for balanced living

· Cultivating healthy habits

· Creating a supportive environment

Chapter 7

Navigating Dietary Trends

· Fad diets: What works and what doesn't

- Making informed Dietary choices

- Sustainable Nutrition for Long-Term Health

Conclusion

Appendix: Resources and References

Description:

Vibrant Vitality"

offers practical guidance, research-backed facts, and realistic tactics for reaching and maintaining optimal health. It also teaches you how to live a balanced, mindful life that results in a better and more fulfilling life.
This book is your compass, pointing the way to a life full of vigor and well-balanced nourishment. Welcome to "Vibrant Vitality: Fuel Your Body, Nourish Your Soul." Finding a sustainable route to well-being might seem like a difficult undertaking in a world full of constantly changing health trends and contradicting information.
In the rush of modern life, it's easy to forget the substantial impact that lifestyle choices have on overall health. "Vibrant

Vitality" offers a comprehensive perspective that goes beyond calorie counting and restricted diets in an attempt to demystify the complexities of healthy living. Our goal is to give you the knowledge and abilities you need to develop long-lasting well-being, not just help you achieve a temporary state of health.

Within the pages of this book, you will find the dietary knowledge, mindfulness practices, and holistic health methods that are the cornerstones of a flourishing existence. We will explore the intricacies of a balanced diet, ponder the transformative power of mindful eating, and learn how mental, emotional, and physical health are all interconnected. This book is not just a compilation of data; it's a practical guide filled with manageable exercises, delicious recipes, and lifestyle tips that you can simply implement into your daily routine.

"Vibrant Vitality" is designed to meet you where you are and assist you in achieving your wellness goals, regardless of your level of experience with health. Together, we'll cut through the clutter and adopt a balanced, enjoyable, and sustainable approach to eating well and leading healthy lives. "Vibrant Vitality" is your trustworthy guide as we navigate the sea of health advice and nutritional trends; it offers evidence-based insights, busts myths, and empowers you to make wise decisions.

Are you ready to embark on a journey that goes beyond quick fixes and diets? "Vibrant Vitality" invites you to rediscover the joy of mindful living, nourishing foods for your body, and designing a lifestyle that not only preserves but also enhances your vitality. Begin your journey, and may this book be your guide to finding the vibrant, version of yourself that has always existed.

Introduction

• **Welcome to Vibrant Vitality**

As you embark on this journey of discovery, you will discover a plethora of information, practical insights, and workable strategies that enable you to fuel your body and nourish your soul. Thank you for joining the vibrant journey toward well-being that is "Vibrant Vitality." This book is your guide to unlocking the mysteries of a healthier and more fulfilling life.

In a world where health advice can be confusing and often contradictory,

"Vibrant Vitality" is a reliable resource that helps you cut through the noise and embrace a holistic approach to health. The journey's central theme is the interconnectedness of physical, mental, and emotional well-being, and each chapter is thoughtfully written to give you the knowledge and skills you need to cultivate long-lasting vitality.

Whether you are a seasoned health enthusiast or you are just beginning to pay attention to your health, "Vibrant Vitality" is designed to meet you where you are. It includes everything from mindfulness exercises to holistic health methods, delectable recipes, and realistic lifestyle ideas.

· Let "Vibrant Vitality" be your guide to vibrant living. Savor the recipes, get started, and embrace the lifestyle changes that resonate with you. "Vibrant Vitality" is more than just a book; it's an invitation to rediscover the joy of nourishing your body, mind, and soul. Let's get started! Here's to a journey of health, vitality, and a more vibrant you!

· **Navigating the path to well-being**

The journey to well-being requires a thoughtful and purposeful attitude. "Vibrant Vitality" recognizes that the path to health is intricate and involves many aspects of our lives. Let's look at the key components of this path to well-being:

1. Establishing Your Position:

• Begin by defining your goals and desires for your well-being. What does a healthy, active life look like to you? Knowing where you're headed provides direction for your next steps.

2. The Perspective on Holistic Health:

• Take a holistic approach to health that recognizes the interdependence of the mind, body, and spirit. Being well-rounded involves more than just physical health; mental and emotional equilibrium are equally significant aspects that contribute to your overall vitality.

3. Assessing Current Practices:

• Assess your current lifestyle practices, including how you eat, exercise, sleep, and manage stress. Understanding where you are in your health journey can help you identify areas for improvement.

4. Setting Reasonable Objectives:

• To stay motivated and keep your focus on the bigger picture, divide your well-being goals into attainable benchmarks that you can acknowledge as you go.

Acquiring Information:

• Learn about mindfulness, nutrition, and lifestyle practices. Understanding the science behind well-being helps you make informed decisions and navigate the overwhelming amount of available health information.

6. Bringing About Intentionality:

• Practicing gratitude, growing in self-awareness, and living in the present moment all contribute to a good mindset that supports overall vitality.

Mindfulness is a useful tool for attaining well-being.

7. Building Support Systems:

• Create a network of individuals who share your health aspirations to create a caring environment that will promote responsibility and development.

Alternatively, ask friends and family for assistance.

8. Adjusting to Shift:

• Recognize that the path to well-being is a dynamic one that may require diversions at times. Be flexible in the face of new information, evolving goals, and unpredictable circumstances.

With "Vibrant Vitality," you may view your journey toward well-being as an ongoing process of self-improvement and self-discovery. May each step you take on this path bring you one step closer to leading the vibrant and vital life you deserve.

Chapter 1: Foundations of Vibrant Living

· Understanding Holistic Health

Here is a closer look at the components that make up holistic health. Holistic health is a way of looking at health that considers the connections between different facets of a person's life and recognizes that physical factors are not the only ones that affect health. It includes the state of the mind, body, and soul and emphasizes the integration of these components for overall vitality.

The Body-Mind Connection

• Mental, emotional, and spiritual well-being can have a significant impact on physical health and vice versa. Holistic health acknowledges the close relationship that exists between the mind and the body. It is widely accepted that practices like mindfulness, yoga, and meditation can promote this mind-body synergy.

2. The state of the body:

• Three fundamental elements of overall vitality are a well-balanced and nutritious diet, regular physical activity, and appropriate rest. Physical health is a key part of overall well-being and involves things like food, exercise, sleep, and preventative care.

3. Mental and emotional well-being: Emotional and mental health are vital components of holistic health. Stress management, good relationships, and emotional problem resolution all contribute to a balanced mental and emotional state. Counseling, therapy, and stress-reduction techniques are commonly employed.

4. Spirituality and What Its Goal Is:

• Developing a spiritual element, whether via spiritual activities, meditation, or time spent in nature, may increase overall life satisfaction and contribute to a sense of fulfillment. Holistic health recognizes the relevance of spiritual health and a life purpose.

5. Social and environmental factors: The social and environmental context in which an individual lives also influences holistic health. Healthy living environments, community involvement, and supportive relationships all contribute to well-being. Individuals can create a conducive atmosphere for health by understanding the impact of social and environmental factors.

6. Promotion of Health:

• The cornerstone of holistic health is preventive care, which sees screenings, routine examinations, and early intervention as essential components in detecting and addressing any health concerns before they worsen.

7. Lifestyle Decisions:

• Making deliberate, well-informed decisions that promote overall well-being objectives is the foundation of a sustainable and well-balanced lifestyle. Lifestyle decisions related to diet, exercise, and stress reduction are crucial to holistic health.

To fully comprehend holistic health, one must recognize the intricate relationships between these elements and how each one fits into the overall scheme of well-being. "Vibrant Vitality" is committed to supporting you along this holistic path by providing you with the resources you need to develop health in a comprehensive and integrated manner.

• The Interconnectedness of mind, body and soul

An understanding of this interconnectedness is necessary to cultivate a harmonious and balanced life. The mind, body, and soul are woven into the fabric of human existence in the following ways. The interconnectedness of mind, body, and soul is a fundamental principle of holistic health, acknowledging that these three aspects of an individual are inextricably linked and that they all contribute to overall well-being:

The Body-Mind Connection

The bidirectional relationship between the mind and body is highlighted by practices like biofeedback, meditation, and mindful movement. The mind and body are not separate entities; they constantly influence one another. Physical well-being can affect mood and cognitive function, and emotions, thoughts, and mental states can affect physical health.

2. How Emotions Affect Health: Wholesome health requires recognizing and addressing emotional issues. Conversely, happy feelings and a sound

mind support physical well-being. Persistent stress, worry, or unresolved emotions can manifest as physical ailments.

3. Physical and Spiritual Wellness:

• Exercise and mindful movement are popular because they have the potential to improve spiritual awareness and connection in addition to their physical benefits. Physical health is not only about physical well-being; it also influences spiritual well-being.

4. How Spirituality Affects Mental Health

• Spiritual practices have a significant impact on mental health. Engaging in activities that bring one a sense of meaning, purpose, and connection to something greater than themselves can improve mental resilience and emotional well-being.

5. Leading A Mindful Life:

Being fully present in everyday activities generates a level of awareness that extends to all aspects of life.

Mindfulness, a practice that is grounded in the present moment and emphasizes the interconnectedness of mind, body, and spirit, fosters a holistic approach to well-being.

6. Integrating Holistic Approaches:

• Holistic health approaches often involve practices that address the mind, body, and soul at the same time. Some examples of these practices are spiritual growth, holistic diet, and meditation. These practices all contribute to overall well-being.

7. Life Force and Vitality:

• Many cultural and spiritual traditions emphasize the interdependence of the mind, body, and soul through concepts like life energy, chi, or prana. Acupuncture and energy healing methods aim to balance and improve the flow of this life energy for general health.

Understanding and respecting the interconnection of mind, body, and soul is a fundamental component of the holistic approach promoted in "Vibrant Vitality." This knowledge enables people to cultivate a comprehensive and integrated lifestyle that supports not only physical health but also mental and spiritual well-being. May you find the deep harmony that comes from taking care of every part of your being as you set out on your journey.

• Settling the stage for lasting vitality

"Setting the Scene for Lasting Vitality" refers to building a solid foundation for long-term health and well-being. This foundational stage is the starting point for your journey toward a healthy, vibrant existence. The key elements of establishing the scene for lasting vitality are as follows:

1. Outlining Your Goals and Principles:
• Begin by considering your values and health goals. What matters most to you? Understanding your core values and establishing clear health goals provide you with a purpose that may guide your decisions and actions.

2. Developing a Welfare Objective:
• Visualize the vibrant, active life you desire. Imagining yourself engaging in happy activities, feeling energized, and enjoying general well-being is one of the best methods to establish the circumstances for lasting vitality.

3. Creating a Positive Attitude
• Maintain an optimistic attitude. Your mentality and beliefs around health have a significant impact on your ability to achieve long-lasting vitality. See challenges as opportunities for growth and approach your path to well-being

with an eye on advancement rather than perfection.

4. Choosing to Adhere to Sustainable Practices:

• Make sustainable lifestyle decisions that align with your goals and values. Whether it's prioritizing self-care, working out frequently, or adopting a balanced diet, choose practices that you can truly live with over time.

5. Acknowledging Balance:

• Maintaining a balanced lifestyle—a balanced approach to work, relationships, and leisure—means avoiding extremes and finding a middle ground that supports your overall well-being.

6. Constructing Hardiness

• Recognize that setbacks and disappointments are an inevitable part of any health journey. • Build resilience via life lessons, adaptability while pursuing your goals, and flexibility.

7. Giving Yourself Enough Attention:

• Make self-care a priority and an essential part of your routine. Engaging in pleasurable, relaxing, and rejuvenating activities daily is necessary to maintain mental, emotional, and physical well-being.

8. Establishing a Supportive Environment:

• Surround yourself with a network of friends, family, or community members who share your health objectives. A positive, encouraging environment may provide the accountability and encouragement you need to succeed on your path to better health.

9. Learning More:

• Stay informed about health-related topics. Having information helps you make informed decisions about your lifestyle, nutrition, and exercise routine. Lifelong learning is a key component of building a foundation for long-term vitality.

10. Respecting Progress:

• Acknowledge and celebrate your little accomplishments along the way. Several tiny triumphs encourage positive habits and spur you on to keep moving in the direction of well-being.

As you embark on your journey to enduring vitality with "Vibrant Vitality," consider this foundational stage as a necessary first step toward creating a long-lasting and fulfilling life. May it pave the way for a journey filled with strength, courage, and a profound sense of well-being.

Chapter 2: Nutrition Wisdom

• **Macronutrients and micronutrients: The Essentials**

Understanding macronutrients and micronutrients is necessary for a balanced and nutrient-dense diet that supports overall health and vitality. Let's review the basics of macronutrients and micronutrients.

1. Lipids
• Function: Essential for hormone and enzyme production, tissue growth and repair, and immunological response.
• Sources: Fish, meat, poultry, dairy products, legumes, nuts, and seeds.
2. Carbs and Sugars
• Function: The primary energy source for the body, supporting mental and physical activity.
• Whole grains, legumes, fruits, vegetables, and foods high in starch are sources.
3. Fat on Body:

• Function: Provide a concentrated source of energy, support cell structure, aid in the creation of hormones, and ease the absorption of food.

• Almonds, nuts, avocados, dairy products, fatty fish, and olive oil are among the sources.

Micronutrients: Essential for Maximum Well-Being and Health

1. Vitamins

• Function: Play a crucial role as cofactors in a variety of metabolic processes that support immunity, blood coagulation, and other processes.

• Sources: fruits, vegetables, whole grains, dairy products, and lean meats.

2. Minerals:

• Function: They are necessary for the synthesis of red blood cells, fluid homeostasis, neuron function, and bone health.

• Sources: Leafy green vegetables, dairy products, whole grains, nuts, and seeds.

3. H2O

• Function: Crucial for preserving water, nutrients, body temperature, and overall cellular health.

• Sources: meals that contain a lot of water as well as plain water.

Balancing Macronutrients for Optimal Health:

1. Protein

Aim for a diverse range of essential amino acids by ingesting animal and plant-based protein.

2. Carbs and Sugars

• When it comes to complex carbohydrates, give wholesome foods like fruits, vegetables, and whole grains a higher priority than processed foods and refined sweets.

3. Fat on Body:

• Incorporate healthy fats, such as monounsaturated and polyunsaturated fats, from foods like avocados, almonds, and fatty fish, as well as modest amounts of saturated and trans fats.

Optimizing Micronutrient Intake:

1. Vitamins

• Eat a colorful selection of fruits and vegetables to provide a wide range of vitamins. Consider seasonal and locally sourced foods for freshness and diversity.

2. Minerals:

• Eat a well-balanced diet that includes a range of whole foods to obtain essential minerals; if required, take supplements, but nutrient-rich meals should always come first.

3. Absorption of Water:

• Steer clear of sugar-filled drinks and excessive caffeine throughout the day, and drink enough of water to keep hydrated.

Understanding the roles that macronutrients and micronutrients play in your body's overall health and vitality will help you create a diet that not only satisfies your hunger but also supports it; "Vibrant Vitality" will further assist you in creating a nutrient-dense, well-balanced eating plan that is tailored to your specific needs.

• Building a well-balanced plate

Incorporating a variety of nutrients into your plate ensures that your body gets all it needs to function at its best. Here's how to balance your plate to maintain overall health and vigor:

Place vibrant veggies on half of your plate:

• Vegetables are rich in vitamins, minerals, fiber, and antioxidants; choose a variety of colors to offer a wide range of nutrients. Vegetables include leafy greens, cruciferous vegetables, bell peppers, tomatoes, carrots, and more.

2. Add Lean Meats:

• Lean protein sources include fish, poultry, tofu, lentils, eggs, and lean meat cuts. For variety, consider plant-based protein substitutes. Proteins are necessary for immune system function, muscle regeneration, and overall body upkeep.

3. Employ Whole Grains:

• Choose whole grains: These include fiber and a range of minerals; whole grains release energy gradually and promote sustained vigor. Examples of whole grains are brown rice, quinoa, whole wheat, barley, and oats.

4. Include Healthy Fats:

• Eat fatty fish, nuts, seeds, avocados, olive oil, and almonds in moderation to support brain function, hormone synthesis, and nutrient absorption.

**5. Observe Serving Dimensions:

• Utilize smaller plates and pay attention to your body's signals of hunger and fullness. Adjust serving sizes based on your age, activity level, and overall health goals to avoid overindulging.

6. Limit Sugar-Added Foods and Processed Foods:

• Wherever possible, choose whole, unprocessed meals; processed foods and those high in added sugars can cause inflammation, low energy, and other health issues.

7. Keep Your Hydration Up:

Water is necessary for digestion, nutrition transport, and overall cellular function. Eat meals high in water, such as fruits and vegetables, and drink lots of it throughout the day. Limit sugary drinks and excessive caffeine intake.

8. Assess Your Nutritional Needs:

• Tailor your plate to your specific nutritional needs, accounting for any dietary intolerances, allergies, or health issues you may have. Consult a physician or nutritionist for personalized advice.

9. Intentional Consumption Patterns:

• Cultivate a mindful eating habit that focuses on digesting food thoroughly, savoring every bite, and paying attention to your body's signals of hunger and fullness. This will prevent overindulgence and promote a healthy connection with food.

10. variation & Moderation: - To ensure a broad range of nutrients, embrace variation in your diet. Moderation is crucial since it allows you to partake in a variety of meals without feeling excessively restricted.

You may create a plate that is both nutritionally balanced and satisfies your body's needs by incorporating these ideas into your regular meals. "Vibrant Vitality" will also assist you in making choices that will promote your body's long-term nourishment and health.

• **Unmasking Nutrition myths and fads**

In the always-changing field of nutrition advising, busting common misunderstandings and clearing the air on nutrition fads are essential. In this article, we do just that by dispelling common myths and providing clarity on nutrition fads, enabling you to make well-informed dietary decisions that support your overall health.

1. Myth: Carbs Are the Enemy
• Fact: The body requires complex carbohydrates, which come from whole grains, fruits, and vegetables, to function; refined sugars and processed foods should be eschewed in favor of complex carbohydrates.

2. Myth: There Is No Good Fat
• Factual statement: Good fats come from foods like avocados, almonds, seeds, and olive oil. Lower your diet of

saturated and trans fats and raise your intake of unsaturated fats, which are essential for hormone production, brain function, and nutrition absorption.

3. Myth: Missing meals results in weight loss

The Truth: Eating regular, well-balanced meals keeps your energy levels stable; missing meals can mess with your metabolism, deplete your body of nutrients, and make you more likely to overeat later.

4. Myth: Gluten Is Not Safe for Everyone:

The Truth: For most individuals, whole grains—including gluten—may be a healthy part of a diet; gluten is only a problem for those who have gluten sensitivity or celiac disease.

5. Myth: Low-calorie diets help the body become purer:

The Truth: Excessive detox diets can lead to harm and vitamin deficiencies, but a balanced diet supports the body's natural detoxification processes, which are handled by the kidneys and liver.

6. Myth: Eating fat makes you fat

• Reality: Maintaining a healthy weight does not always come from eating healthy fats in moderation. Rather, weight regulation is determined by the overall balance between energy expenditure and calories consumed.

7. Myth: Not Everyone Requires Supplements of Protein:

• Factual statement: While protein is essential, most people can obtain all the protein they require from a balanced diet; athletes, for example, require additional protein to meet their high protein needs.

8. Myth: Every Food With The Label "Natural" or "Organic" Is Beneficial:

• Factual statement: Focus on full, less processed meals; products labeled "natural" or "organic" do not always imply that they are healthy; processed organic snacks may still be high in sugar and unhealthy fats.

9. Myth: Consuming food after midnight causes weight gain

• Fact: When gaining weight, focus more on the overall amount of calories ingested and burned than the type and quantity of food consumed during the day.

10. Myth: One-Size-Fits-All Diets Work:
- Reality: Age, activity level, and health issues all affect an individual's nutritional needs, which is why personalized nutrition planning is preferable to following a set diet plan.

11. Myth: Superfoods Are the Cure-All - Truth: While nutrient-dense foods are beneficial, there is no one "superfood" that can address every health issue. Instead, a diversified, well-balanced diet is necessary for overall welfare.

"Vibrant Vitality" will help you navigate the complex world of nutrition and establish a sustainable, balanced approach to eating well by busting myths and fads around nutrition. This will empower you to make decisions based on scientific evidence and your own unique needs.

Chapter 3: Mindful eating

· **The art of mindful consumption**
This intentional process of selecting, cooking, and eating food is called the

"art of mindful consumption." We can improve our overall state of well-being, deepen our relationship with our bodies, and enjoy food more when we incorporate mindfulness into our eating practices. Here's how to embrace the art of mindful consumption:

1. Living in the moment:

• Begin your meal by taking a moment to savor your food's tastes, textures, and colors. During the dining experience, engage all of your senses and permit yourself to be present.

2. Eliminate Distractions:

• Set up a specific area for meals, switch off technology, and minimize outside distractions so that you may focus fully on the food and its flavors.

3. Bite Firmly:

• Dice food slowly and well, not just to aid in digestion but also to fully enjoy each meal's flavor and texture.

4. Recognize Your Hunger and Fullness:

• Be mindful of your body's cues about hunger and fullness. Eat when you're hungry and stop when you're satisfied. Don't eat in a rush.

5. Make Sense of Everything:

• Pay attention to the flavors, textures, and colors of your food. Eating with your whole body enhances the sensory experience and strengthens your bond with the meal.

6. Know When to Eat Without Feeling:

• Be conscious of your emotions and the reasons behind your hunger. Mindful eating is recognizing emotional cues and refraining from using food as a sole coping mechanism.

7. Express Thank You:

• Express gratitude for the nourishment you receive from food. Consider the journey food takes to reach your plate. Develop an understanding of the connection between food and life.

8. Being Aware of Portion Sizes

• Pay attention to portion sizes and serve yourself reasonable amounts; pay attention to your body's signals instead of overindulging out of habit or peer pressure.

9. Choose Nutrient-Rich Foods:

• Pay attention to the nutritional value of the meals you select, emphasizing a balance of macro- and micronutrients; select foods that promote overall health and your body's requirements.

10. Slow Down: - Eat mindfully, taking your time, so that your body has enough time to register fullness and fully enjoy the flavors of your meal.

11. Mindful Cooking: - Incorporate mindfulness into the process of preparing meals. Cook with attention, relishing the ingredients and the labor of love.

12. Practice awareness: - Practice mindfulness throughout the day by monitoring your eating habits, drink preferences, and overall nutritional

patterns. This may be done outside of mealtimes.

The art of mindful consumption invites you to approach eating with awareness, appreciation, and presence. By incorporating these practices into your daily life, you can transform the act of eating into a nourishing and fulfilling experience that supports your overall well-being. "Vibrant Vitality" will guide you further on this journey of mindful living and nutrition.

• Cultivating a healthy relationship with food

A healthy relationship with food requires a positive, mindful, and balanced approach to eating. You can transform your relationship with food by creating a deeper connection with it and intentionally nourishing your body. Here is a guide to assist you on your journey to a mindful and healthy relationship with food:

Develop the practice of mindful eating:

• To help you appreciate eating more, practice mindfulness as you eat. Chew slowly and savor every mouthful, taking in the flavors, textures, colors, and scents of your meal.

2. Be Aware of Your Body:

Eat just when you are hungry and stop when you are full. Avoid eating because you are bored, stressed out, or feeling any other unpleasant emotion. • Pay attention to your body's signals of hunger and fullness.

Avoid following rigid diets:

• Give up on tight diets and focus on giving your body a variety of wholesome meals. • Create a balanced, sustainable eating plan that meets your nutritional needs.

4. Give in to Intuitive Cooking:

• Trust your body. Eating intuitively is listening to your body's cues and satiating your feelings of hunger and fullness instead of blindly adhering to external guidelines or restrictions.

5. Let Go of the Remorse:

• Practice self-compassion. Acknowledge that a single meal does not define your overall health. Let go of guilt regarding the meals you chose. Take note of how your eating habits are balanced overall.

6. Respect the Diversity of Foods:

• Take pleasure in the diversity of flavors, textures, and cultural influences in your meals and eat a wide variety of foods to ensure that your diet contains a wide range of nutrients.

7. Bust Common Myths About Food:

• Explore and challenge societal and cultural perceptions of food and body image. Accept what your body feels good and is healthy.

8. View Food as Fuel and Pleasure:

• Recognize that food is a source of enjoyment and nourishment for your body. • Find a balance between giving your body nutrient-dense meals and occasionally indulging guilt-free in sweets.

9. Get your food ready and cook it:

• Participate actively in meal preparation. Cooking is a creative and entertaining activity that may enhance your relationship with the food you eat.

10. Put Your Health First: Make lifestyle decisions that promote overall health rather than weight in place of unreachable body objectives.

11. Seek Professional Assistance: - You may choose to seek assistance from a therapist, registered dietitian, or other medical professional if you struggle with eating disorders or have a negative relationship with food.

12. Practice Self-Reflection: - Analyze your relationship with food regularly. -

Find out how different meals affect you physically and emotionally. - Adjust your plan based on what's best for your overall health.

Developing a positive connection with food requires conscious choices, self-compassion, and self-awareness. "Vibrant Vitality" will assist you in developing a long-term, holistic nutrition plan that supports your general health and well-being.

• Savoring the flavor: mindful eating practices

The artwork "Savoring the Flavor: Mindful Eating Practices" encourages you to fully engage with your meals, appreciating the sensory experience and fostering a deeper connection with your food. These mindful eating techniques will help you enjoy dining while promoting a healthy relationship with food.

1. Begin by expressing gratitude:

• Take a moment before you start eating to express your gratitude for the food that is in front of you and to think about how it got there.

2. Comprehend Everything:

Using your senses to prepare your body and mind for a meal involves paying attention to the flavors, textures, colors, and overall appearance of the food.

3. Bite Firmly:

• Chew mindfully, gently, and with awareness of the flavors and textures of your food. This enhances digestion and allows you to thoroughly enjoy the flavor of every bite.

4. Place Your Cutlery Down:

• You may also try eating more slowly and deliberately, enjoying every piece by occasionally putting down your utensils in between portions.

5. Consume Food Without Diversion:

• Turn off technology and set up a special space for meals. By eliminating outside distractions, you can focus fully on the eating process and savor the flavor without feeling pressured in a lot of ways.

6. Savor Every Bite:

• Approach each bite with gratitude, acknowledging the labor-intensive process that went into preparing the meal as well as the sustenance it provides for your body.

7. Mindful Portion Control:

• Give yourself reasonable serving sizes so that you may enjoy each meal without overindulging and focus on the food's quality rather than its quantity.

8. Pay attention to your body:

• Throughout your meal, take a minute to check in with your body and gauge how full and hungry you are. By doing this, you will develop the ability to listen to your body's signals instead of those coming from outside sources.

9. Willfully Consume:

• Eat with awareness. Avoid mindless snacking or eating out of habit. Choose and enjoy meals that contribute to your health goals.

10. Play with Flavors: - To embrace diversity in your meals, add herbs, spices, and seasonings to your food to make it taste better. This will help each meal be a new experience.

11. Mindful Drinking: - Be mindful of the beverages you have with your meals. Steer clear of sugary drinks that might overpower the flavor and instead choose water or other hydrating beverages that complement your meal.

12. Review Your Experience: - Once you've consumed your food, take a moment to reflect on the emotional and physical feelings it brought you. This type of self-reflection helps you become

more conscious of and connected to your eating habits.

"Savoring the Flavor: Mindful Eating Practices" is an ongoing journey of cultivating awareness and appreciation for the food you consume. By incorporating these practices into your daily meals, you can transform eating into a mindful and pleasurable experience that nourishes both your body and soul. "Vibrant Vitality" will further assist you in integrating mindfulness into your nutrition for long-lasting well-being.

Chapter 4: Holistic Health Practices

• Exercise for energy and well-being

Here is a guide on exercise for energy and well-being. Exercise is a strong tool for boosting energy levels, improving mood, and promoting overall well-being. Completing a regular physical activity program may have many great impacts on your physical and mental health.

1. Choose Activities for Getting Pleasure:

• Engage in activities you enjoy. Whether it's yoga, hiking, cycling, or dancing, picking things you love to do increases the likelihood that you'll stick with them.

2. Start with attainable objectives:

• Start with modest and doable objectives and set reachable milestones to help build confidence and cultivate a positive connection with exercise.

3. Integrate Cardiovascular and Strength Training:

• Include both aerobic exercises (such as walking, running, or cycling) and strength training. Aerobic exercises strengthen your heart, while strength training increases muscle strength and metabolism.

4. Prioritize consistency over intensity:

• Consistency is the key to reaping the benefits of exercise; even short, regular sessions can have positive effects.

Regular activity is more helpful than intense, occasional activities.

5. Be Aware of Your Body:

• As your fitness level rises, gradually increase the intensity and duration of your workouts. • Pay attention to your body's signals. If you start to feel weary, take a break. Overexerting yourself can result in injuries or burnout.

6. Schedule Regular Exercise Time:

• Prioritize physical exercise in your daily schedule and schedule time for it, whether it be in the morning, at lunch, or night.

Examine Mind-Body Activities: In addition to its physical benefits, mind-body activities such as yoga or tai chi can aid with stress alleviation and mental wellness.

8. Get Outside: Take advantage of outdoor activities. Getting some fresh air and natural light may boost mood and energy levels. This may be achieved by

taking a walk in the park or going on a hike in the woods.

9. Stay hydrated: Staying well-hydrated before, during, and after exercise can help you perform at your peak and prevent fatigue.

10. Include Flexibility and Stretching Exercises: To enhance range of motion, reduce tight muscles, and enhance general flexibility, incorporate stretching and flexibility exercises into your routine.

11. Locate Exercise Partners: - Join a group fitness class or work out with friends. Social support, accountability, and encouragement may be obtained by belonging to a community or having a workout partner.

12. Make relaxation and recovery a priority: - Allow your body to rest and recover. Sleeping sufficiently and taking days off between intense workouts are

essential for preventing burnout and improving overall health.

13. Set realistic Expectations: - Recognize that the benefits of exercise may not be immediately obvious. Set realistic expectations and focus on how your mood, energy level, and overall health will improve.

14. Experiment with Different Modalities: - See what works best for you when it comes to exercising. Cross-training offers many benefits and may liven up your routine.

Regular exercise improves mood, vitality, and overall well-being; "Vibrant Vitality" will assist you in creating a personalized fitness plan that suits your needs and advances your journey toward long-term health.

- **Stress management strategies**

Effective stress management is essential to maintaining overall well-being.

Chronic stress can have detrimental effects on your physical and mental health, so learning coping strategies that promote resilience and relaxation is essential. Here are some daily stress-reduction techniques:

1. Practice Deep Breaths:

• Use deep, diaphragmatic breathing methods to help activate the body's relaxation response. Breathe in deeply with your nose, hold it for a little while, and then slowly exhale through your mouth.

2. Mindfulness-based meditation:

• Incorporate mindfulness meditation into your daily practice. Mindfulness meditation entails focusing on the present now while being aware of your breath, sensations, and surroundings. It can reduce stress and enhance emotional well-being.

3. Regular Exercise:

• Engage in regular physical activity. Endorphins, the body's natural stress relievers, are released when you walk, run, perform yoga, dance, or engage in other physical activity.

4. Establish a Timetable:

• Create a daily timetable that delineates precise times for work, relaxation, and self-nurturing. A scheduled routine reduces uncertainty and anxiety.

5. Put Your Sleep First:

• Make sure you get enough sleep each night because not getting enough sleep might make you more stressed. Prioritize relaxation, create a nightly routine, and create a pleasant sleeping environment.

6. Establish reasonable goals:

• Divide tasks into smaller, more doable tasks and establish realistic goals. • Prioritize your projects and focus on what is achievable rather than overwhelming yourself with an extensive to-do list.

7. Social Connection:
• Maintain your social connections with friends and family. By discussing your thoughts and emotions with others, you may build a sense of community and get emotional support from others.
Limiting Agents: **8
• Reducing or avoiding stimulants such as caffeine and nicotine, particularly in the few hours before bed, since these medications may increase anxiety and impair sleep.
9. Quit Using Technology:
• Take breaks from electronic devices, especially social media and work-related communication. • Set limits for screen time to reduce information overload and promote relaxation.
10. Practice Relaxation Techniques: - Try out a variety of relaxation techniques, such as guided imagery, progressive muscle relaxation, or aromatherapy. Determine which ones

suit you the most, then include them in your daily routine.

11. Laugh and Have Fun: - Laughing is a natural method to relax. Engage in joyful pursuits, watch comedies, or spend time with people who make you laugh.

12. Express gratitude: - Make it a practice to reflect on the positive events in your life. Gratitude may assist you in shifting your focus from issues to the positive aspects of your day.

13. Seek professional Support: If stress becomes too much to bear, consider seeking assistance from a mental health professional. Therapy, counseling, or support groups can provide guidance and coping methods.

14. Learn to Say No: - Establish boundaries and learn to say no when necessary. Overcommitting can lead to increased stress and burnout. Prioritize your health and make time for self-care.

Combining these methods will help you become more resilient and more skillful in handling life's challenges. Stress is a natural part of life, but how you respond to it greatly affects your general health. "Vibrant Vitality" will provide additional guidance and insights on leading a resilient, well-balanced lifestyle.

• Quality sleep: The foundation of vitality

great sleep is fundamental to overall vitality and well-being. Regular sleep patterns are linked to physical health, cognitive performance, and emotional resilience. The following advice will assist you in prioritizing and making great sleep the cornerstone of your vitality:

1. Adhere to a Sleep Schedule:
• Create a regular sleep schedule that includes weekends. By keeping your

body's internal clock in check, this will improve your quality of sleep.

2. Create a Calm Sleep Schedule:

• Create a bedtime routine that includes reading, mild stretching, or listening to soothing music to help your body realize when it's time to rest.

3. Create the Ideal Sleep Environment:

• Create a comfortable and sleep-friendly environment. Ensure that your bedroom is dark, cold, and quiet. Invest in a comfortable mattress and pillows to promote restful sleep.

4. Cut Down on Screen Time Before Bed:

• Minimize the amount of time you spend using devices before bed since the blue light they produce can interfere with the body's normal production of the hormone melatonin, which regulates sleep.

5. Think About Your Food and Drink Choices:

• Avoid heavy meals, caffeine, and large amounts of liquids just before bed. If you're hungry, eat a little snack and choose calming beverages like herbal tea.

6. Take Up Frequent Exercise:

• Regular exercise will ensure that you complete your workout at least a few hours before going to bed, which will improve your quality of sleep.

7. Manage Your Tension:

• Before going to bed, use stress-reduction techniques like progressive muscle relaxation, deep breathing, or meditation to calm your mind.

8. Pay attention to the surroundings where you sleep:

• Invest in a comfortable mattress and pillows that support good posture while you sleep; regularly replace your bedding; and have a clutter-free, immaculate bedroom.

9. Establish a Wind-Down Time Before Sleep:

• Create a bedtime routine that helps you unwind and de-stress; avoid bright lights and stimulating activities an hour before bedtime.

10. Minimize Naps: If you do take naps throughout the day, try to keep them to no more than 20 to 30 minutes. Avoid taking long or late afternoon naps as they might interfere with your nighttime sleep.

11. Pay Attention to Your Sleep Position: - Although it's usually recommended to sleep on your back to maintain spinal alignment, choose a position that works best for you.

12. Address Sleep Disorders: - Consult a physician if you have difficulty falling asleep regularly. Certain interventions or treatments may be required for sleep disorders such as sleep apnea or insomnia.

13. Limit Stimulants: Reduce your intake of stimulants like caffeine and nicotine, especially in the hours before bed, to avoid sleep problems brought on by these substances.

14. Monitor Your Light Exposure: - Try to obtain as much natural light as you can during the day, especially in the morning. - In the evening, turn down the lights to signal your body that it's time to unwind.

Making quality sleep a priority is essential to maintaining vibrant health and vitality. "Vibrant Vitality" provides further details and advice on how to optimize your sleep routine for optimal wellness

Chapter 5: Recipes for Wellness

• Energizing Breakfasts

Here are some wholesome and energizing breakfast ideas to get your mornings going: Consuming a substantial and wholesome breakfast supplies essential nutrients and long-lasting energy, which creates a positive energy balance for the rest of the day.

1. Greek yogurt parfait:

• Top Greek yogurt with honey, granola, and fresh berries for a hearty and energizing breakfast that's rich in antioxidants, fiber, and protein.

2. Nut Butter Banana Oatmeal:

• Cook oats in milk or water, then top with banana slices and a generous dollop of nut butter (which adds healthy fats and protein to the complex carbohydrates).

3. Avocado toast with a poached egg:

• Spread mashed avocado over whole-grain toast and top with a perfectly poached egg for a balanced combination of fiber, protein, and healthy fats.

4. Smoothie Bowl:
• Add your favorite fruits, leafy greens, and a liquid base (yogurt or almond milk) to the blended smoothie. Pour the smoothie into a bowl and top with granola, sliced fruit, almonds, and seeds for added flavor and nutrition.

5. Pancakes with whole-grain berries:
• Top pancakes made with whole grain flour with fresh berries; the antioxidants, vitamins, and minerals in the berries combine with the long-lasting vitality of whole grains.

Chia Seed Pudding

6*To make a nutrient-dense, energy-boosting breakfast, whisk together chia seeds with milk or plant-based milk substitute and refrigerate overnight. The following morning, top with almonds, fruits, and honey.

7. Vegetable and Egg Breakfast Wrap:
Eggs, your favorite vegetables, and a whole-grain tortilla topped with cheese

make up this breakfast that combines essential nutrients, fiber, and protein.

8. Quinoa in Breakfast Bowl: Because it is a complete protein, quinoa is a filling and nutrient-dense option. To finish, prepare some quinoa and toss in some Greek yogurt, sliced almonds, and fresh fruit.

9. Peanut Butter Banana Bread: Top whole-grain bread with peanut butter and banana slices to get a mix of complex carbohydrates, protein, and healthy fats.

10. Cottage Cheese and Fruit Bowl: - provide your favorite fruits (berries, pineapple, or kiwis) to cottage cheese to provide natural sweetness and vitamins. Cottage cheese also provides protein.

11. Vegetable Omelets: - In addition to eggs, which provide protein, add a variety of vegetables, such as bell peppers, tomatoes, spinach, and mushrooms, to your colorful omelet to provide fiber and essential nutrients.

12. DIY Breakfast Burrito: -Scrambled eggs, black beans, chopped tomatoes, and cheese are piled on a whole-grain tortilla for flavor and antioxidants. Try experimenting with different combinations of these energizing breakfast ideas to see what works best for your palate and dietary needs to support your energy levels throughout the morning. "Vibrant Vitality" will provide additional guidance on how to create a nourishing and well-balanced diet to enhance your overall health.

• Nourishing Lunches and dinner

You must feed your body wholesome, well-balanced meals if you want to sustain energy and promote overall well-being. Here are some ideas for satisfying lunches and dinners that contain a variety of nutrients:

1. Grilled salmon served with quinoa and roasted veggies:
• Grill salmon fillets to serve over cooked quinoa, and then roast a colorful side dish consisting of a variety of vegetables, such as bell peppers, cherry tomatoes, and asparagus.
2. Chickpeas and veggies stir-fried:
• Serve over brown rice or quinoa, and add a fragrant sauce made of ginger, garlic, soy sauce, and sesame oil. Sauté chickpeas with a range of colorful vegetables, such as broccoli, carrots, and bell peppers.
3. Feta and Spinach Stuffed Chicken Breast:
• Stuff feta cheese and spinach mixture into butterfly chicken breasts; bake until cooked through, and serve with green beans and roasted sweet potatoes on the side.
4. Lentil and vegetable soup:

• To make a hearty and aromatic lentil and vegetable soup, combine lentils, carrots, celery, tomatoes, and spinach. For added flavor, add herbs and spices.

5. Shrimp and Avocado Salad:

• Toss shrimp with cherry tomatoes, fresh greens, and a light vinaigrette dressing; this salad is rich in protein, healthy fats, and vitamins.

6. Quinoa and black bean bowl:

• In a bowl, mix cooked quinoa, black beans, corn, chopped tomatoes, and avocado for a nutrient-dense, light dinner. Top with a lime-cilantro vinaigrette.

7. Vegetable and turkey skewers:

• Thread cubed turkey, bell peppers, zucchini, and cherry tomatoes onto skewers; bake or broil until done, and serve with whole-grain couscous on the side.

8. Chickpeas with sweet potatoes in a curry:

• Serve sweet potatoes, chickpeas, and spinach over brown rice or quinoa in a coconut milk-based curry for a hearty and nourishing supper.

9. Baked Cod with Lemon and Herbs: - Combine olive oil, lemon juice, and fresh herbs with cod fillets and bake until flaky. For a full dinner, pair with quinoa and steamed broccoli.

10. Tofu with Vegetable Stir-Fry: Mix bright vegetables such as bell peppers, carrots, and snow peas with tofu and stir with soy ginger or teriyaki sauce before serving over brown rice.

11. Mediterranean Chickpea Salad: Toss chickpeas with cucumber, cherry tomatoes, red onion, olives, and feta cheese. Toss with olive oil, lemon juice, and herbs for a light and refreshing option.

12. Roasted Spaghetti Squash with Tomato and Basil Sauce: Top with grated Parmesan cheese for a hearty,

low-carb twist on spaghetti. Drizzle with homemade tomato and basil sauce.

Try experimenting with different ingredients and flavor profiles to create meals that cater to your taste preferences and dietary needs. These nourishing lunch and dinner ideas offer a variety of nutrients, including protein, fiber, vitamins, and minerals. "Vibrant Vitality" will provide additional insights into creating balanced and nourishing meals to support your overall well-being.

· Irresistible snacks and smoothies

Nutrient-dense snacks and smoothies may be made deliciously. Here are some ideas for delicious and nutrient-dense snack and smoothie ideas:

Appetizing Snacks:

1. Slices of banana with nut butter:

• Spread almond or peanut butter on banana slices for a satisfying and nourishing snack. Top with chia seeds for extra texture and protein.

2. Hummus with veggie sticks:

• Dip bell pepper, cucumber, and carrot sticks into hummus for a crunchy, high-protein snack. Hummus is a great source of plant-based protein and good fats.

3. Greek yogurt parfait:

• Top Greek yogurt with granola, berries, and honey to create a delicious and high-protein parfait; feel free to add your favorite nuts and fruits.

4. Mix Trail:

• To meet your demands for both sweet and savory, whip up a batch of trail mix, which is a great on-the-go snack made of nuts, seeds, dried fruits, and dark chocolate chips.

5. Apple slices with almond butter:

• Cut apples into slices and serve them with almond butter (you can also add a little cinnamon for flavor) for a great combination of fiber, vitamins, and healthy fats.

6. Cubes of cottage cheese and pineapple:

• Try this cool snack of fresh pineapple cubes and cottage cheese; the sweet, tropical pineapple goes nicely with the protein-rich cottage cheese.

7. Rice Cake with Avocado and Cherry Tomatoes:

• Top a rice cake with cherry tomatoes and mashed avocado for an easy and satisfying snack. Add a dash of salt and pepper.

8. Dark Chocolate Almonds:

• Toss almonds with a small quantity of dark chocolate for a tasty treat; dark chocolate provides antioxidants and healthy fats, while almonds provide protein.

9. Sushi rolls with vegetables:

• Roll nori, avocado, cucumber, and julienned carrots into small sushi rolls and serve with soy sauce for a refreshing and crunchy snack.

10. Edamame Pods: Boil the pods and sprinkle with sea salt; edamame is a terrific plant-based protein source and a satisfying and healthful snack.

Alluring Smoothies:

Berry Smoothie Blast:

Blend mixed berries, bananas, Greek yogurt, and a tiny bit of almond milk to make a refreshing, powerfully antioxidant smoothie.

2. Green Goddess Smoothie:

• Blend spinach, kale, pineapple, banana, and coconut water to create a nutrient-dense green smoothie; squeeze in some lime for taste.

3. Tropical Paradise Smoothie:

• Blend mango, pineapple, coconut milk, and a small handful of spinach to create a tropical-inspired smoothie; add shredded coconut as a garnish for extra flavor.

4. Peanut butter and chocolate protein smoothie:
• Blend almond milk, peanut butter, banana, and chocolate protein powder to create a silky, high-protein smoothie.
5. Peach and ginger smoothie:
• For a zesty, refreshing smoothie that boosts immunity, mix yogurt, orange juice, peaches, and fresh ginger.
6. Cucumber Mint Cooler Smoothie:
• Blend cucumber, mint leaves, lime juice, honey, and Greek yogurt into a cool, hydrating smoothie.
7. Smoothie of Avocado Bliss with Blueberries:
• Blend spinach, avocado, blueberries, and coconut water into a luscious smoothie that's high in antioxidants and nutrients.
8. Smoothie with bananas and coffee:
• Brew a strong cup of coffee, then add banana, almond milk, and a scoop of

protein powder to produce a potent and energizing smoothie.

9. Pineapple Coconut Chia Smoothie: Pineapple, coconut milk, chia seeds, and a tiny bit of honey are blended to create this tropical, high-fiber smoothie.

10. Oatmeal Cookie Smoothie: To create a smoothie that tastes like oatmeal cookies, blend oats, almond milk, banana, cinnamon, and a tiny bit of vanilla extract.

Here are some ideas that you can tweak to suit your tastes and dietary requirements. "Vibrant Vitality" will provide more information on how to build a nourishing and well-rounded diet to support your overall health. These tasty snacks and smoothies have a range of tastes, textures, and nutrients to keep you full and energized all day.

Chapter 6: Life Style Strategies

· **Time management for balanced living**

Consciously organizing and planning around work, personal responsibilities, and self-care leads to a meaningful and balanced existence. The following time management strategies can help you achieve balance in your life:

1. Establish Task Priorities:

• Using your values and objectives as a guide, prioritize your most important tasks into lists that will help you carve out time for the things that truly matter.

2. Create a Schedule:

• Make a daily or weekly plan that includes designated times for work, personal commitments, and self-care. Consistency is built by diligent adherence to your schedule.

3. Establish reasonable goals:

• Divide more difficult tasks into smaller, more doable steps. Set reasonable daily or weekly goals. These actions will prevent burnout and provide you with a sense of accomplishment.

4. Strengthen Your Refusal Skills:

• Overcommitting may lead to stress and hinder your ability to effectively manage your time. Establish limits and find it easy to say no when necessary.

5. Assign Tasks:

• Delegate as much as you can, both at work and at home. This allows people to feel empowered and frees them up to focus on other vital tasks.

6. Group-Related Assignments: Organize similar tasks into batches and complete them in the designated time slots to minimize mental hopping and increase output.

7. Use the Pomodoro Technique:

• Use the Pomodoro Technique to work on a task for 25 focused minutes (a

Pomodoro), then take a 5-minute break. After four Pomodoro, take a longer break. This will enhance productivity.

8. Reducing Disruptions:

• Minimize distractions when working intensively. Make your workstation quiet, turn off unnecessary notifications, and close tabs that aren't being used to increase focus.

9. Deviations from the Timetable:

• Make time in your schedule for regular breaks. These little respites help you stay focused and prevent burnout. Use them to stretch, take a quick walk, or engage in mindfulness exercises.

• **Cultivating healthy habits**

Creating and upholding healthful routines in several aspects of your life might be a life-changing experience that improves your general state of well-being. The following are useful strategies to help you do this:

1. Start Small: Set realistic goals that will help you build confidence over time and lay the foundation for larger gains.

2. Give One Habit Your Whole Attention: Don't try to change several habits at once; instead, concentrate on one behavior at a time. Once it becomes ingrained, you may go on to the next.

3. Clearly State Your Goals: Establish SMART (measurable, achievable, relevant, and time-bound) goals for your habits. Having well-defined goals will enable you to track your development and stay motivated.

4. Establish a routine: Make sure your healthy habits are part of a routine. Repetition improves habits until they become more automatic.

5. Anchor Old Habits to New Ones: Link the new habit and everyday routines or activities you currently perform. This will help you remember the new

behavior by associating it with something you regularly do.

6. Use Visual Aids: Post messages or other objects that act as visual signals to assist you in creating the habits you want. Place visual cues or reminders in prominent areas.

7. Create a Network of Assistance:

• Share your goals with friends, family, or coworkers who can encourage and support you. Having a support system increases motivation and responsibility.

8. Honor Little Victories: Congratulate yourself on your little accomplishments along the way. This will boost your confidence and positive conduct.

9. Incorporate Variability: To prevent boredom and increase the likelihood of continuous adherence, use an innovative strategy to uphold your good behaviors.

10. Practice Mindfulness: Pay attention to details and be present in the moment while you go about your everyday

business. This can help you become more conscious of your environment and make thoughtful decisions that are beneficial to your health.

11. Learn from Your Mistakes: Rather than viewing setbacks as failures, acknowledge that they are inevitable and make use of the opportunity to improve your approach.

12. Make sleep a priority: To improve overall health, make obtaining a good night's sleep a priority by creating a regular sleep pattern and a cozy resting space.

13. Maintain Hydration: Staying properly hydrated is essential for many bodily functions and improves overall health. Make sure you are drinking enough water throughout the day.

- **Creating a supporting environment**

Fostering overall well-being and success necessitates building a supportive environment. Whether at work, home, or in your community, a supportive environment may positively affect your mental, emotional, and physical health. Here are some strategies to help you develop a pleasant atmosphere.

1. Cultivate Positive Connections: Surround yourself with people who are encouraging, understanding, and uplifted by you. Cultivate connections that improve your wellness.

2. Have Open Communication: Promote the expression of opinions and sentiments as well as candid and open communication in your interactions to foster an environment where everyone feels heard and understood.

3. Set Boundaries: Communicate your requirements and boundaries to others. Respect the boundaries that others have set. Set healthy boundaries that provide a

supportive environment. Set boundaries that are clear to protect your well-being.

4. Encourage Collaboration: Foster a culture of collaboration and teamwork in both personal and professional settings. When individuals come together to accomplish common goals, a feeling of support and belonging is generated.

5. Honor accomplishments: Promote an environment where people's efforts and successes are valued and acknowledged, and celebrate and honor accomplishments of all sizes.

6. Offer Helpful Criticism: Encourage personal growth and progress while maintaining a supportive atmosphere by offering constructive criticism politely and positively.

Chapter 7: Navigating Dietary Trends

• Fad diets: What works and what doesn't

This is an overview of some popular fad diets, with an emphasis on what works and what doesn't: Fad diets often promise rapid weight loss or better health, but many of them are unsustainable, deficient in vital nutrients, and harmful to the user's health.

1. Ketones found in diet:
What Works: The high-fat, low-carb, moderate-protein ketogenic diet has been shown to help treat several illnesses, including epilepsy, and may help some individuals lose weight, especially in the short term.
What Doesn't: Constipation, the "keto flu," and an elevated risk of heart disease if the diet is high in unhealthy fats are among the negative effects of a strict ketogenic diet, which may eventually lead to nutritional deficiencies.

2. The Paleo Lifestyle:
What Works: The Paleo diet emphasizes whole, unprocessed meals that focus on fruits, vegetables, lean meats, nuts, and seeds while avoiding processed foods and refined sugars.
• What Doesn't: It might be challenging to stick to the diet for a prolonged length of time. Strictly excluding specific food groups may result in nutrient deficiencies. Experts dispute how historically true the diet's idea is.
3. Intermittent Fasting:
• What Works: According to research, alternating periods of eating and fasting may assist in encouraging weight loss, improve metabolic health, and maybe even prolong life.
• What Doesn't: It might not be optimal for everyone, and adherence could be challenging. Some people might feel angry, weary, or overeat during non-fasting times.

4. Detoxification diets:
• What Works: Short-term detox diets can help cut out processed foods and encourage the consumption of whole, nutrient-dense meals.
• What Doesn't: Juice cleanses and other extreme detoxification methods might leave you deficient in vitamins and are not long-term fixes. There is a lack of scientific evidence to support many detox diets, and claims made about "cleansing toxins" are often untrue.
5. Low-Fat Diet:
• What Works: When dietary fat intake is slightly decreased, especially saturated fats, replacing harmful fats from sources like nuts, seeds, and avocados with healthier fats may help improve heart health.
• What Doesn't work: Instead of strictly restricting total fat intake, focus on the quality of fats. Diets that are extremely low in fat may not be sustainable and

may leave a person with insufficient intake of essential fatty acids.

6. Plant-Based Diets:

• What Works: Eating a diet rich in fruits, vegetables, and whole grains, whether vegetarian or vegan, may help regulate weight and enhance cardiovascular health.

• What Doesn't: A haphazard plant-based diet may leave you short in B12, iron, and omega-3 fatty acids, so it's important to make sure you're receiving enough of these nutrients from plant-based sources or supplements.

7. Gluten-Free Diet:

• What Works: A gluten-free diet is necessary for those who have celiac disease or gluten sensitivity.

• What Doesn't: There's no evidence that a gluten-free diet promotes health in individuals without gluten-related conditions, and if it's not well planned, it may leave you deficient in some nutrients.

8. Alkaline Diet:

• What Works: Emphasizing meals rich in foods that generate an alkaline environment, such as fruits and vegetables, can promote a diet rich in essential nutrients.

• What Doesn't: Tight dietary restrictions on acidic foods might result in nutritional imbalances, and there is no scientific evidence to support the theory that diet may alter body pH.

Fad diets are frequently linked to health risks and lack long-term sustainability; instead, focus on a balanced and varied diet that includes a wide range of nutrient-dense foods. Consult with a healthcare provider or a registered dietitian before making significant dietary changes, especially if you have underlying health conditions. "Vibrant Vitality" will offer evidence-based guidance on maintaining a well-balanced and sustainable approach to nutrition.

• Making informed Dietary choices

You need to make intelligent food choices to promote overall health and wellness. The following basic concepts will assist you in making well-informed nutrition decisions:
Stressing Whole, Unprocessed Foods:
• Make complete, unprocessed meals a priority whenever possible. These foods are rich in essential nutrients and promote overall health. Fruits, vegetables, whole grains, lean meats, and healthy fats should be prioritized.
**2. Balancing Macronutrients:
• Ensure that the macronutrients in your meals are well-balanced. Aim for a combination of proteins, lipids, and carbohydrates to support various bodily functions and provide sustained energy.

**3. Give Preference to Plant-Based Foods:

• Consume a diverse array of plant-based foods. Fruits, vegetables, legumes, nuts, and seeds are good sources of antioxidants, fiber, and nutrients.

**4. Keep an Eye on Your Eating:

• Indulge in meals with pleasure, watch portion sizes to avoid overindulging, and pay attention to your body's hunger and fullness cues.

**5. Keep Your Hydration Up:

• Drink enough water throughout the day. Water is essential for proper digestion, hydration, and overall bodily functions.

6. Limit Sugar-Added Foods and Processed Foods:

• Reduce the quantity of processed foods and beverages that have a lot of added sugar. These foods and beverages are often deficient in nutrients and can lead to health issues.

7. Add Nutritious Fats:

• Include foods high in heart-healthy fats (olive oil, almonds, avocados, and fatty fish) in your diet. These fats help your body absorb nutrients and sustain heart health and brain function.

Select Whole Grains

8. opt for whole grains rather than processed grains. Whole grains, such as brown rice, quinoa, and whole wheat, are higher in fiber and minerals.

9. Change Up the Sources of Your Protein: Consume a variety of high-protein meals, including fish, poultry, eggs, legumes, dairy products, lean meats, and plant-based alternatives like tempeh and tofu.

10. Read nutrition labels carefully: To help you make informed decisions, learn how to read nutrition labels on packaged items and be sure to take notice of serving sizes, ingredient lists, and nutritional value.

• Sustainable Nutrition for Long-Term Health

Sustainable nutrition for long-term health requires making decisions that support environmental health as well as personal health. The following principles and practices will assist you in adopting a sustainable and health-promoting approach to nutrition:

1. Prioritize Whole, Plant-Based Foods: Plant-based foods are rich in fiber, antioxidants, and essential nutrients. Include a variety of fruits, vegetables, legumes, nuts, and whole grains in your diet to highlight a plant-based diet.

2. Choose Eco-Friendly Proteins: If you consume animal products, choose ethically raised, sustainably produced, and wild-caught varieties. You may also choose sustainable protein sources like tempeh, tofu, beans, and plant-based substitutes.

3. Include Seasonal and Local food: Whenever possible, focus on seasonal and local food; this supports regional farmers, reduces the environmental effect of shipping, and ensures that meals are fresher and higher in nutrients.

4. Decrease food Wastage Mindful meal planning, purchasing, and storage are all crucial practices to help minimize food loss. You can also decrease food waste by finding creative ways to use leftovers, composting food scraps, and keeping an eye on expiration dates.

5. Choose Sustainable Fish: To preserve the health of ocean ecosystems, choose seafood that has been responsibly caught by looking for certificates like MSC (Marine Stewardship Council).

6. Admit Old and Complete Grains:

• Consume a diet high in whole grains and ancient grains, such as farro, quinoa, and barley; these grains are nutrient-dense and have little effect on the environment.

7. Wherever Possible, Choose Local and Organic: Prioritize nutrient-dense foods above strictly adhering to organic labels to reduce pesticide exposure and support environmentally friendly agriculture practices.

8. Mindful Eating Practices: By eating consciously, which includes appreciating each meal, eating slowly, and paying attention to signs of hunger and fullness, you may cultivate an appreciation for the nutrition that food provides.

9. Hydrate Sustainably - Use reusable water bottles, use locally and sustainably sourced beverages, store single-use plastics, and make sustainable beverage choices.

10. Promote the adoption of environmentally friendly farming practices:

Learn about and lend support to regenerative and sustainable agricultural methods that prioritize soil health and minimize their detrimental effects. impacts on the ecosystem and contributes to sustaining food security.

Conclusion

Vibrant Vitality" emphasizes the connections between sustainability, mindfulness, and nutrition to provide you with a complete strategy for making choices that promote your long-term health, vitality, and the health of the world. It leads you on a transforming path toward overall health and well-being.

This book covers a lot of territory, from understanding the fundamentals of nutrition to creating a caring atmosphere, selecting a sustainable diet, and forming healthy habits. By adopting complete, unprocessed meals, balancing macronutrients, and prioritizing plant-based alternatives, you are not only giving your body the nourishment it needs but also contributing to a more sustainable and ecologically responsible lifestyle.

You've learned how being present in your daily life may enhance your connection with food, reduce stress, and foster a positive perspective.

Mindfulness is a common theme throughout "Vibrant Vitality." These habits are essential to living a healthy and full life, as are stress management strategies and prioritizing enough sleep.

The subtleties of sustainable nutrition have also been covered in the book, and you are encouraged to consider the environmental impact of the foods you eat. By choosing food that is locally sourced, in season, and sustainably produced, you can support regenerative agriculture and contribute to a better future for future generations.

Creating a supportive atmosphere, choosing prudent foods, and forming healthy behaviors are ongoing tasks. As you continue on your journey toward robust health, remember the importance of self-compassion, balance, and adaptability. Every person's health is connected to the health of the community and the earth.

A guidebook called "Vibrant Vitality" will enable you to make choices that uphold your moral principles and result in a fulfilling, sustainable, and lively existence. The concepts offered in this book will assist you in beginning the journey toward holistic well-being, regardless of your objectives—whether they are to increase your energy, lessen stress, or just take care of your body and mind.

Cheers to a life of harmony, meaning, and good health; may your journey to vigorous vitality be filled with happiness, development, and a strong feeling of self-connection to others and to this wonderful planet we call home.

Appendix: Resources and References

1. Dan Buettner's book "The Blue Zones: Lessons for Living Longer from the People Who've Lived the Longest":
• Examines the living habits of the communities with the greatest life expectancies globally to provide insights on longevity and well-being.

2. The book "The Power of Now" by Eckhart Tolle
• A guide to mindfulness and living in the present that can help you achieve a deeper level of awareness and peace.

3. The book "How Not to Die" by Michael Greger, MD:
Examines the relationship between nutrition and the prevention and treatment of chronic diseases, providing evidence-based suggestions for a plant-based diet.

4. The book "Atomic Habits" by James Clear:

• Offers realistic techniques for creating and breaking habits, enabling you to improve your daily life.

5. "Braiding Sweetgrass: Indigenous Wisdom, Scientific Knowledge, and the Teachings of Plants" by Robin Wall Kimmerer:

• Fosters a stronger connection with nature by combining scientific understanding with traditional knowledge.